HealThySelf
(Heal-Thy-Self)

7-Day Guide to
Starting Your Weight Loss Journey

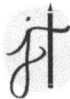

JT Publishing House

Published by JT Publishing Spartanburg, South Carolina
www.jtpublishinghouse.com

JT Publishing House books and products are available through most bookstores. To contact JT Publishing House, visit www.jtpublishinghouse.com.

Library of Congress Cataloging-in-Publication Data
Jackson, S. Fanchon.

HealThySelf: 7-day guide to starting your weight loss journey
Fanchon Sade Jackson
pages cm 96

ISBN 978-1-7341793-4-7 (paperback) – ISBN 978-1-7341793-5-4 (ebook)

Printed in the United States of America 10 9 8 7 6 5 4 3 2 1

Dedication

What makes a hero?

Heroism is defined as the ability to face adversity fearlessly, and it is knowing there will be plenty of wins and failures.

You know how to make a little become a lot when there's more mouths to feed than cans in your cupboard.

I dedicate this work to my Granny, Jean, and my Grandmother, Rose, my two superheroes.

To my heartbeats, thank you for allowing mommy to be Fanchon! There will be days where you don't feel like yourself, you won't feel like you are enough, but listen to mommy, I want you to know you are more than enough. I love the three of you with all my heart, and I'll always be here.

To my beautiful butterfly, Grace, I love you.

Foreword

Discipline. Courage. Results!

Discipline is not just the ability to remain committed, it's the dedicated choice to stick with it, over, and over, and over again—even when everything suggests, points in the direction of, and mandates that you travel down Easy Street! It's courage.

Courage is the decision not to face the giant, but the little things that tell us where we are, or what we have is all we deserve. It's getting up and doing what we don't want to do. It's being honest with ourselves. It's about rolling away the stone, facing what stinks, and what seems impossible to revive.

But, if we develop discipline and clinch on to courage, we get results.

Results are the dream, the desires of our hearts, the manifestation of what discipline and courage produce.

Sade, results were inevitable.

The courage it took to face you, is not only admirable but inspiring.

Few actually make the investment in themselves and do the hard work to see what's on the other side!

My purest hope for the results of your work is that it ignites discipline and courage in others.

Jossalyn Wilson, MSOD
www.jossalynwilson.com
Author, Executive Coach

By the Day

Allow Me to Introduce Myself

Who am I?

Fanchon Sade Jackson.

I can almost guarantee my name was mispronounced in your head, or you gave a little smirk as to why my mom might have given me my name.

Well, my uncle named me actually.

Now that my name is out of the way, it is important to tell you why I'm here, in this space.

I'm here, writing because I wish someone would have written to me.

I wish someone would have written to me so I could have been further along in life and my weight loss process.

Perhaps you've had some doubts about "another" weight loss book, but this one isn't the same, which you've also likely heard. But really, it isn't.

I believe my journey holds value in helping you start your journey because I'm the lady you've passed in your local grocery store or market.

I'm a daughter, a soccer mom to three children, and a divorcee.

I'm the mom who doesn't fold laundry until a few days later (because I don't have it all together), and I'm a loyal friend.

Yes, I'm her!

Now maybe, just maybe, you've found or currently find yourself wearing one, or possibly more of those hats.

I applaud you!

I applaud you on everything you've done thus far, and mom to mom, friend to friend, *thank you!*

I've worn way too many of those hats at one time, and I became incapable of balancing my life to sustain myself mentally, spiritually, emotionally, and physically.

I failed me!

I failed at loving who I was because of what the commercials projected, the latest trends dictated, or what housewives were supposed to "be."

I failed to become me.

I put too much emphasis on what I should be, rather than my current state.

I'll share more details as we go along, so there's a clear understanding of how I got there—you know, *"there."*

My Journey

One of my favorite quotes comes from Buddha, "To enjoy good health, to bring true happiness to one's family, to bring peace to all, one must first discipline and control one's mind. If a man can control his mind, he can find the way to Enlightenment, and all wisdom and virtue will naturally come to him."

I love that quote because one's mind has to be able to think its way out of things, even when it comes to your health.

I grew up thinking that I am the way that I am due to genealogy.

I looked at what I saw around me and believed as I grew older, I'd have to deal with heart disease, diabetes, or high blood pressure.

They (people) have said because it runs in my family, I may have at least one diagnosis.

However, I refuse to believe or accept that message. Although, in the beginning, my actions confirmed that I would write a similar life story as my family members.

Over the past two years, I have started a journey. Yes, another journey, but not your typical weight loss journey. I started the journey where I decided to make a lifestyle change that would affect those around me, as well as impact my healing.

My highest weight was 320 pounds, that's when I made up my mind to change. As I write, I weigh 207 pounds.

In this book, I hope you develop some takeaway messages from my journey.

It's not waking up every morning at 4:15 am and going to the gym, it's not the sacrifices you make when choosing a salad over a burger, it is about being at peace within and knowing that what you choose is just that, a choice.

I have a choice whether or not I want to make the best decisions as it relates to my health.

Some say it takes 21 days to gain a habit.

I say it starts with seven days of consistency.

Often, we make choices for everything else, but neglect the decisions about our health because we assume we will be here long enough to make a different choice at some point.

Each year, over 2 million people around the world die from obesity, the thought of that amazes me.

Obesity is not bias!

It does not care about race, age, gender, or geographic location.

From America to South Africa, obesity cripples people, as one of the leading causes of death among the human race.

Therefore, I want to share my journey with you, what I'm doing, and what I've done that will hopefully help you kickstart your journey to better living and better health.

Remember, you matter!

Don't allow anyone to place their negative opinions over you. You are worthy of complete wholeness spiritually, mentally, and physically.

Allow me to introduce myself.

I'm Fanchon Sade Jackson, the woman

who decided to heal-thy-self!

Before we begin...

Throughout these pages, you'll have a chance to write down your next goal, and what you would like to change about yourself.

There will also be sections that allow you to pause, and some parts have deliberate actions that will enable you to repeat an affirmation.

Use those moments to display vulnerability, be real with where you are in your journey.

Allow yourself time to digest every chapter and engage deeply.

Here's your first repeat! Repeat after me,

"I'm a work in progress, and I will allow myself time to heal."

Day One: Self "ish"

Repeat This:
"So what if this is day one again!"

Day one can, at times, be draining because there are high expectations related to what you are no longer putting up with, or no longer wanting. So many different thoughts can plague your mind.

I'm sure you've either thrown away all of your snacks or visited the store to buy some lettuce.

Yes, lettuce!

Imagine someone asks you for gourmet lettuce. Funny, right?

Seriously, we've all had a lot of *day ones*.

My day one was the day after my ex-husband left me.

Although it wasn't about my weight, there was a part of me that thought, well maybe if I change, he'll notice me.

Pause:
If someone leaves you based on your looks, they were not meant for you!

Yes, I had butt dimples, stretch marks, and rubbing thighs.

Oh, and I dare not forget the line, *"You're so pretty, for a big girl."*

This statement is offensive, so if you have ever uttered those words, please don't say it again.

The individual you are referring to is cute regardless!

I stopped eating, wrong decision!

I wanted instant change!

The "I'll drop 20 pounds in 2 weeks" change, and that just wasn't the right decision—that was my first day one.

Round two of round one began by acknowledging I am who I am because of me, no one else.

I was the common denominator.

I was the reason I was in that specific situation.

My day one was full of tears.

I sat on the couch and said to myself, *"You're big as f!*#!"*

Yes, those exact words.

It wasn't pretty; it wasn't a "let me start

this new regimen" conversation.

It was, *"Sade, you're big as f!*#!"*

I went to the mirror and had a couple of Britney Spears' moments.

I realized that the only way up was to get up!

I didn't have money for the gym, so I started small.

I'm a mother of three.

After taking my children to school, going to work, getting off, picking them up from afterschool, getting home to cook supper, and dealing with the unforeseen whining of the day, I had precisely 9 hours and 27 minutes to myself each night (three of those minutes were used to scream at my children to turn off the lights).

Not to mention that within those hours, I

needed to sleep.

However, I was commited to starting, so depending on the season, I either walked for 30 minutes or an hour.

During that time, I had a lot to talk about with myself.

I realized that exercise is only a small percentage of self-healing.

Exercise gives you the ability to get up and accomplish the established goal, and now that I had my blood pumping, it was time for a change.

With Your Selfish Self

Being selfish allows you to knock down the door of feeling that you are not enough.

You are enough!

Scream it from the top of your lungs, "I am enough!"

I remember having my breaking point.

I was home alone, and I was depressed.

I couldn't get anyone to answer their phone, so I stopped, prayed, and asked the peace of God to overtake my mind and lead me where I should go.

Funny thing, I believe the Lord led me to Hobby Lobby.

I grabbed some paint, paintbrushes, and a canvas.

I didn't know what I was going to do!

Although very creative, I am no Picasso.

I went home and prayed again.

Tears began to flow.

At that moment, I realized everything I faced and experienced needed an outlet.

I needed to let it all out.

Every emotion from anger to sadness, and sadness to joy, I needed to say it.

There are things in our lives that are unable to heal because we never speak it out of our mouths.

For example, when we go to the doctor, one of the first things they say is, "Tell me what's wrong."

You almost diagnose yourself, then you are given something to help you heal.

Everything I felt about myself, the sense of unworthiness, the feeling of shame, I needed to get it out, so I did.

I grabbed the paint, and I started to write out everything I felt.

Without acknowledgment, I covered the 20 x 15 canvas with words.

I poured everything I had on the canvas that day. Then, I painted over the words as I repeated, "I am enough, I am worthy" aloud.

Each color symbolized something I was determined to obtain and achieve.

The color blue signified strength and wisdom, as it has a calming effect.

I associated the color red with power, desire, and love. Green represented life, harmony, safety, and growth, and the colors continued.

Finally, I'd let it all out!

I let out the things I couldn't say, the things that hurt me, and the fear of being alone.

I had my selfish moment.

I took time out for me!

Being "selfish," in this sense, doesn't make you arrogant, it makes you aware that you matter.

Taking back your health is one way of regaining control mentally, physically, and emotioally.

You have the power to change the way you think about yourself and how others receive you.

Now before you make the change, think about why you are changing and make yourself number one on your list.

Pause:
Please do not make drastic changes that you are not willing to make a lifestyle.

One way to start is portion control.

Remember, you are a product of what you eat. Said differently, you are what you eat.

I'm not suggesting you are a cow if you eat a burger.

I'm saying if you eat the half-pound burger with the bun, bacon, lettuce, pickle, onion, cheese, and mayo, you cannot complain when you aren't able to fit into your favorite jeans.

You cannot continue to blame others for what you've done to yourself.

Pause:
Check out the article,
"How Do You Know if You're Full?"
https://www.livestrong.com/article/489875-how-does-your-stomach-tell-your-brain-that-youre-full/

According to *Hunger and Satiety*, an article featured in Living Strong, "the feeling of fullness that tells you to stop eating, are complex functions regulated by numerous feedback mechanisms in your body.

One of those signals comes from your stomach wall stretching to accommodate the meal you are eating.

Nerve stretch receptors send signals to the brain that the stomach is expanding, and you can begin to taper off and stop eating."

To sum up the article, we know when we are full. No one knows your body better than you.

Although we can consume it, it doesn't mean that we aren't already full.

What makes us feel like we have to eat everything in front of us?

Is it the amount of time spent preparing the meal or the price paid for the meal?

Or, is it because the food is right in front of us?

Two: "Saucer it!" If it runs over the saucer, it's too much.

Using a saucer is very helpful when starting your weight loss journey.

We tend to eat way more than what our body is supposed to consume because our eyes see more.

Isn't it funny how we look at our plates and assume it's not enough because we are conditioned to think there should be more food on the plate!

If we continue to live that way, we will never see the glass as half full.

Instead, we will always see it as half empty.

When properly plating a table, there's

more silverware than plates and glasses, but just because there's more silverware that does not mean we have to eat from each fork or spoon during one serving.

Each piece of silverware has a specific use, but we do not use all the pieces during one setting, but we tend to want to eat the full plate when there are more meals to follow.

The saucer method is simple.

Get a smaller plate than what you consider a dinner plate, and make the right decisions.

A well-balanced meal is a protein, a vegetable, and a carb.

If it can't fit in your hand, then it's too much.

Beginning the saucer method requires self-control.

Three: "Eat" A balanced meal

The keyword is "balanced!"

Do not overeat!

In recent studies, a well-planned meal includes dairy, vegetables, fruits, grains, and protein.

While it sounds like a lot of food, it's actually not. However, the amount of food from each group matters.

Most restaurants only offer one side item with an entrée, and like most Americans, we choose the food of substance, which may not be the healthiest choice.

I have found truth in the notion that it is more cost-efficient to buy processed food than it is to buy an apple.

Why does it seem that everything good for us, naturally produced by the earth, is more expensive?

Although the healthier options may cost more, it's important to remember your health is not something you can't afford to sacrifice.

A balanced meal is good for you, and it will help you kick start your journey to a better you.

Day Two: Keep It Private

Repeat This:

"What I eat in private will show up in public."

The Great Announcement

"I'm starting my weight loss journey" (insert echoes and applauds).

In reality, however, you hear crickets, "me too," or even the question, "Isn't this your third time around?" *The nerve of some people.*

Well, maybe this time is your third time around, or possibly your sixth.

Who said there was a race to having good health?

Don't worry. I'll wait!

No one! No one ever said the journey would be thirty days, stop after the weight is gone, or when the goal reached.

Starting is just the beginning.

Let me guess you're waiting on the New Year to kickstart your journey again.

This year will finally be your year, right?

Beloved, New Year's resolutions are for people who are waiting for tomorrow to make decisions about things that could've happened yesterday.

Do not fall for it. Don't put off what you can do today for tomorrow, because tomorrow brings a brand-new struggle and new plans.

The announcement alone can cause doubt, feelings of failure, and it can place you into depression, not loving who you are.

I've made my share of announcements over the years.

After putting the status on Facebook, I immediately looked for "likes" from my peers or the cheers of those who agreed with my journey.

After those three hearts and four likes on Facebook, I was on my way to a better lifestyle for sure.

I was going to prove them wrong.

I was going to show my progress along the way, I was going to give pointers and show the "healthy pictures" of my food. I was hype!

Pause:
You do know I set myself up for failure,

right? Never make a change for you based on the likes or opinions of others.

After day three, I noticed I was becoming exhausted, trying to live up to what I thought people wanted to see.

Before I knew it, I had fewer and fewer likes, and the hearts, well there weren't any hearts.

Then I started telling myself, "I don't have to post it; I'll show them."

It was a setup.

I set myself up for failure by trying to prove others wrong when, in reality, I wasn't prepared mentally to take on the responsibility of being consistent in my journey.

I started to question myself, "How can you lead someone to better health when you can't be consistent with a simple post?"

Consistency is critical, even when no one is watching.

I set myself up for the announcement, little by little, and I started wavering from the decision.

Then, I started having what is commonly called a "*cheat day.*"

A "cheat day" became every day, and I allowed myself to get into a place of no one's watching, and no one cares!

I started to believe losing weigh wouldn't work for me, so I gave up.

Disappointment is the leading cause of failed attempts when it comes to losing weight.

We tend to give up or blame our genetic makeup. Sometimes that notion is correct (it is genetics), but you can break the cycle.

This time around, I'd like to encourage you not to make the announcement.

There is a saying, "big success is won when no one is watching."

If you make an announcement, make a declaration to yourself, "I will never go back."

Make small changes and form the habit of living a better life.

No announcement can beat you truly living your best life—that's inner peace, better health, loving self, loving others, mental stability, and having joy.

Are you tired yet?

Are you tired of starting over?

Are you tired of watching someone else's success story?

Are you tired of thinking you're stuck?

If so, make you self-declaration in private, or between you and me.

There's space below for you to start. I'll go first, and you can finish by declaring it over yourself.

Self-declaration: I will no longer live my life in the shadows of what I could've done. I will look at myself daily, love myself, and encourage myself to move, no matter how I feel. I choose to become who I want to be by making the best decisions for me.

Now it's your turn…

_____
_____
_____
_____
_____
_____
_____
_____
_____
_____
_____
_____
_____
_____
_____
_____
_____
_____
_____
_____
_____
_____

_____

_____

_____

_____

_____

_____

_____

_____

_____

_____

_____

_____

_____

_____

_____

_____

_____

_____

_____

_____

_____

_____

_____

_____

_____

Day Three: It's Me, It's Me Accountability

Repeat This:
"It is all me."

When using the word accountability, I can almost guarantee you thought of someone who could hold you accountable, but not yourself.

Accountability starts with you!

Say this statement aloud, "accountability starts with (Insert your name)."

Now allow that thought to sink in.

How do you feel?

No one can make you do anything; only you have that power.

Almost everything in life is a choice. You choose to get up, go to work, what you eat, and what you wear.

You control the story!

When I started taking my weight loss journey seriously, I started with portion control. I realized I could do the fitness, but I still wanted to eat.

I love food! Who doesn't?

However, I started eating less and throwing my food away after going out to eat.

My friends began to say things like, "You're wasteful!"

"You're not eating," and "you're eating rabbit food."

Trust me; I have heard it all.

The notion that everyone around you will need to adjust to your new lifestyle is far-fetched.

Even your children can and will get on board. If you develop small habits for them in the beginning, they will not depart from it.

At first, the commentary bothered me.

Better yet, it infuriated me because the statements were not true! I ate, I just had to hold myself accountable.

I was also upset because the people making the comments were people who I believed would encourage me.

Guess what?

They were encouraging me.

They believed in me; they were holding me accountable for what I said and what I did.

Listen, you cannot get mad with people for asking, "Hey, aren't you on a diet?"

Those comments are them holding you accountable for what YOU said.

If you ever want people to take you seriously, start following what you say and make your words actions!

Workout partners

I get asked about workout partners all the time, and honestly, my answer would be, "No, don't do it."

I'll tell you my reasons.

Although I've attempted to have a workout partner, it just never seems to work out for me.

You may be "done, done" with how you look or feel about yourself, and your workout partner may not have the same goals.

They might believe in having "cheat days," or they may not see the importance of showing up to the gym every morning at 5:00 am.

It happened to me far more times than I'd like to admit. I had to realize that whether or not I had a partner, I had to get up and go to the gym.

I had to choose to do it for myself; anything less was choosing to fail.

Workout partners have come and gone, but my determination for better health is far more important than a "no call, no show" to the gym.

To sum it up, "*issano*" from me!

However, if it works for you, try it.

Remember, consistency starts with you, not with your partner.

Sometimes writing things out will help you remind yourself of your WHY!

Write down your "why!" It will start to help you follow through on your declaration.

Use the space below to begin to hold yourself accountable to your goals and commitments.

_____
_____
_____
_____
_____
_____
_____
_____
_____
_____

Day Four: Start Day
"Off My A$$"

Truth moment, I wake up at 4:28 am every morning, and I struggle!

Some would say my body should be used to the early morning routine, and I would agree, but it's still a struggle.

I have four other alarms that follow that alarm.

Yes, the struggle.

My morning routine includes the first alarm, which I immediately turn off and pull my covers off of me. And because I embrace my "birthday suit," the cold temperature of the room slowly wakes up my body.

The second alarm sounds at 4:30 am. Yes, two minutes later, because I know how stubborn I can be—accountability.

Don't judge me, the back to back alarms help me.

The second alarm is my final warning. I place my feet on the floor to stand.

There are times I wait for the third alarm, and the extra signal causes me to rush.

I usually work myself into a headache.

I might be a little cranky, forget to put on my workout gloves, or even have my shirt on backward.

By the third alarm (4:45 am), I'm likely grabbing my keys and heading out of the house.

Thankfully, my gym is four minutes away from my home (depending on my speed, I can get there in two minutes).

By the fourth alarm, I'm inside the gym (or should be inside the gym) on a treadmill or the Stairmaster—some form of exercise equipment.

Typically, it takes me three minutes to warm up, and in the spirit of transparency, I'm generally exhausted.

However, I'm off my ass, and it hasn't always been that way for me.

There have been several times when starting my weight loss journey that I chose to stay in bed.

Pause:
Listen to your body. If you need rest
then rest. Do not strain your body,
you'll pay for it later.

Staying in bed is choosing laziness.

Where are you choosing to stay?

If you are not choosing to remain in a complacent state, what are your next steps?

Remember, any step forward is a step in the right direction; you're moving!

At times we talk ourselves out of progress.

We might get up, but then we come up with a million other things to do.

Our progress is based on when we choose to get up.

Start!

Tell yourself mentally and physically what you will and will not allow anymore when it comes to your journey.

Below, there is space to decide what you will allow in your life.

You may not have the time to jot it all down right now, so take your time and come back to this exercise to finish it later.

Start today!

Today I choose... _____

_____

_____

_____

_____

_____

_____

_____

_____

_____

_____

_____

_____

_____

_____

_____

_____

_____

_____

_____

_____

_____

Jackson

_____

_____

_____

_____

_____

_____

_____

_____

_____

_____

_____

_____

_____

_____

_____

_____

_____

_____

_____

_____

_____

_____

_____

_____

_____

_____
_____
_____
_____
_____
_____
_____
_____
_____
_____
_____
_____
_____
_____
_____
_____
_____
_____
_____
_____
_____
_____
_____
_____
_____

Day Five: Opinions "F-it"

Repeat This:
"They will talk, and I will choose when
to listen!"

One of the most significant forms of
warfare on your journey will be the
opinions of others.

"They" will talk until "they" are heard!

What are you going to do?

I'll tell you!

Sit there and listen.

In your mind, analyze everything they are saying about your journey.

They will often attempt to tell you what you should do, what worked for them, why they don't do this or that anymore, and they might even suggest going to the gym with you.

Please do not get discouraged!

Do me a favor!

Before you listen to them, look at them.

Yes, look at them and see what their body says about them.

Looks can be deceiving.

Being skinny doesn't mean the person is healthy or fit. I've met some of the most unfit, lazy, yet skinny people, along my journey.

How much weight have the opinions of others helped you lose this year?

Again, I will wait…

The answer is none!

Other's opinions helped you lose absolutely nothing, so why would you care about what they think is best for you?

I am not suggesting that hearing other's stories or taking notes and nuggets from them won't encourage you.

After all, you're reading mine, and I would like to think that my words will help inflame a fire inside of you to move forward.

However, hearing other people's stories can be overwhelming, and sometimes it can create a sense of impossibility.

Pause:
You are worth starting your journey

At times we have so much we want to change about ourselves that we forget that the one who created us is pleased with His outcome.

The freckles, the mole, the shape of your eyes, and your nose, are God's perfect creation. You are perfect in His eyes.

The greatest opinion is in what you think about yourself.

Do you love yourself?

One of my favorite passages reads, "Love your neighbor as you love yourself."

That passage resonates with me because it suggests that we can't love someone else until we love ourselves.

No one can give complete love until they

love themselves.

When you look in the mirror, what do you see?

Every blemish, every part of your being, is because He (God) created you in His image and for His liking.

God placed you in His hands; He formed you.

Isn't that an amazing confirmation?

The Creator took His time with you, and you are perfect in His eyes.

Self-healing

Self-healing will require you to embrace your thighs. It will cause you to love every stretchmark and love-handle.

When I realized that, I was ready to take over my journey. I looked in the mirror, and I embraced everything about me.

My opinion is what mattered.

What I said about myself mattered.

I chose to change because I wasn't in the best health situation.

I shed many tears because I didn't look like the model or Betty Boop, nor was I shaped like a Coca Cola.

I believed I wasn't good enough.

I would hear what men said or even watched how they looked at women as they walked by, and I felt like I was not enough.

Self-healing requires you to dig deep and understand why you have that opinion of yourself.

I went to counseling for a year and a half.

Every week, I sat in someone's office so I could uncover the things hidden within.

In a community where there are sayings such as, "you're young, you'll get over it," or "you have time to get things right," it's hard to reach out to someone else to help you speak about what others want to silence in you.

Speak up for yourself. If you're hurting, name it!

Ask for help so your healing can begin.

In this space take a moment and name whatever "it" is that's hurting you, and make a declaration over yourself about your ways to heal.

_____
_____
_____
_____
_____
_____
_____
_____
_____
_____
_____
_____
_____
_____
_____
_____
_____
_____
_____
_____
_____

_____

_____

_____

_____

_____

_____

_____

_____

_____

_____

_____

_____

_____

_____

_____

_____

_____

_____

_____

_____

_____

_____

_____

_____

_____

Day Five

Day Six: Eat the Cookie

Repeat This:
"It's just a cookie!"

Sounds unhealthy, right?

Let it sink in.

Eat the cookie. Yes, that cookie!

Too many times, we get caught up in the "I can't eat that" mindset.

There's a quote I love; it reads, "We are drawn away by our desires."

Meaning, if we desire it, we're going to do whatever "it" is.

So, go ahead, eat the cookie!

In the previous chapter, I shared a little about portion control (not dieting), but it's simply you controlling the amount of food you put in your body.

Ultimately, I believe we give up way too easily.

There are times I have given up too easily. I let the cookie overtake my mind, and I believed there was no coming back from my indulge.

Does indulging mean you're a failure?

Does one cookie set you back for the entire day?

Putting too much emphasis on failure creates an open door for failure to sail into the room.

I'm frequently asked about calorie

counting.

Calorie counting is good if it works for you. I can not tell you if it is going to work or not. Do what works for you.

Pause:
Stop starting things to lose twenty pounds in five days. You are setting yourself up for failure, ultimately starting your day one all over again.

Eating a cookie does not equate to an unhealthy lifestyle.

An unhealthy lifestyle is not taking control over what you put in your body. I can't express to you how much eating a "cookie" is not a failure.

You fail when you give up.

Giving up is NOT an option. You've come way too far to give up.

I can remember the first time I gave up.

Yes, I gave up!

It was January 15, 2017, a date I will never forget.

That is the day my emotions got to me— the day of my angel's birthday.

In 2010, I lost my child, Grace. She was stillborn.

Every year when the day comes around, I'm overwhelmed emotionally. It hits me like a mountain of bricks. I find myself eating more and talking less.

My emotions get the best of me.

Grieving can cause you to do things that you say you'd never do, and my "I would never" was overeating.

It wasn't just a cookie; it was all of my

comfort foods. I ate all the foods that would help me feel full enough to go to sleep—emotional eating! *#MyStruggle*

Emotional Eating

It is crazy because so many things happened throughout the year that "should" have caused me to overeat, but I resisted. I have self-control at all times, except on that day.

I can't control how sad, angry, and unworthy, I feel on that day.

Nor can I fully articulate how food comforts my emotional space, pretending it is the best way to cope.

As a mother, not hearing the sweet cry of my child was and is the most difficult thing for me to move past.

Having no control over losing her, I constantly fight to not inflict harm against myself.

Perhaps grieving is not your trigger.

Maybe it is you feeling unworthy, not qualified, or overlooked, or possibly, you are and have always been the black sheep of your family.

Maybe someone hurt you unimaginably, *I'm sorry*.

Whatever it is, I cannot express how much <u>YOU</u> matter.

The moments that attempt to drive you to emotional eating will emerge, and we never know how strong it will affect us.

Emotions are described as a natural, intuitive state of mind.

Suggesting, if I think my way out of it, I can accomplish or overcome anything, even emotional eating.

Jackson
76

Overcome

I have tried several methods to help me stablize my emotions.

I have tried self-help groups, meditation, and counseling, all of which served a purpose and helped me process.

I honestly owe my life to my counselor, Molly.

When I decided to talk and become whole, I found this thing that most would likely compare to happiness, but it is not happiness alone. I found the combination of great pleasure and happiness—*pure joy*.

I learned that I find joy in knowing things change, and things do not remain the same.

Yes, something tragic happened in my life, but I will overcome it.

I will fight to live!

It is not just my physical body; my mental state also needs continued conditioning and renewal.

Some of the most significant battles occur in our mind long before it manifests in the earth.

Stop living in your mind and start fighting for a better day and a greater tomorrow.

Please put down the fork and work to identify the root of your emotional eating habits.

Remember, putting too much emphasis on failing will opens the door to failure.

A cookie is just that, a cookie, it is not a pound or five pounds.

Instead, it is knowing deeply that the cookie is your choice. It is not controlled or determined by anything else.

Develop personal accountability.

So, I ask, "Who took the cookie from the cookie jar?"

Pause:
Reflect on what encouraged you to make your decisions. Here's your moment to let it out, and remember nothing is wrong with taking and/or eating the cookie!

_____
_____
_____
_____
_____
_____
_____
_____
_____
_____
_____
_____
_____
_____
_____
_____

_____

_____

_____

_____

_____

_____

_____

_____

_____

_____

_____

_____

_____

_____

_____

_____

_____

_____

_____

_____

_____

_____

_____

_____

_____

Day Six

Day Seven: Show Your A$$

Repeat This:
"I'm becoming!"

Once upon a time, I felt inadequate and incapable of reaching my goal look. I took pictures, normally of my front and back side, and marked the areas where I wanted to see improvement.

I suggest doing something similar if you want to consistently track your progress.

You may not get there in 7 days, 21 days, or 365 days, but you are slowly progressing to become the person you desire.

Show yourself, I mean why not?

You did it.

Yes, you may have had some help along the way but, you did it!

No one creates something to hide it.

You did not wake up and go to the gym to hide yourself.

Maybe crop tops are not your thing (just yet), but at least you can fit into those jeans again.

Seriously, I hope that you are starting to feel and see your insecurities drifting away.

On a previous day, I said being skinny doesn't mean you are healthy, and getting fit does not mean everyone will applaud you.

However, you have come too far to not show off your progress.

Although sometimes unseen, it doesn't matter how big or small it is, the fact is that you aren't who you were in the beginning.

Go ahead and show yourself off.

You are slowly becoming who you want to become, and it is not easy.

I do not want you to feel like the past several days are a 7-day miracle to better health or being slim thick.

This journey hopefully encourages you to know you matter.

You have the final say about what goes in and comes out of you.

Your inner beauty should radiate so much that it appears on the outside.

Day Seven

You are redefining who you are mentally, physically, and emotionally.

My desire and hope for you is that you take this book and make it your own story.

Your story won't be like mine, and it shouldn't.

Seven days of reflecting and getting to know who you are on the inside and outside I hope will help you see that it takes more than you just getting up and going to a gym.

It takes more than you making an announcement to the world.

It takes more than someone holding you accountable.

It takes more than what you put in your body.

It takes a made-up mind and complete

consistency in what you want for yourself.

When you choose to live and have a better life and stop giving up on yourself, that's when you start embracing your "day one."

Take care of YOU.

Breathe!

Tomorrow will be day 8, keep going!

You have a chance every morning to do the impossible.

We can move our limbs; we can breathe in and out in a rhythm, take delight in knowing that no one else can be you.

No more blaming others for failed diets or accountability.

No more posting announcements without following through with your choices in private first.

No more shaming yourself for not being a size 8.

We go through so much in a day, not to mention a month, or a year.

We will make mistakes, we will cry, we will eat the cookie, but we will also grow and change.

It starts with you!

Here's to a healthier, healed you! Live unapologetically.

Cheers to day eight!

Acknowledgments

To God, my Creator thank you for seeing the things I don't see. Thank you for not allowing me to destroy myself. Thank you for being my Father.

I want to thank my friends for loving me through all of my sizes.

To my 5:00 am crew (Gold's Gym Greer) thank you for motivating me.

To my dear friends (without mentioning all of you) thank you for being that 2:00 am phone call and letting me cry on your shoulders. I know what I gave you and shared with you was heavy. I pray God continues to grant you extra strength for your race. I want you to know and see that

I am better, and it's alright to release what I gave you. I love you guys so much.

To my family, without naming all of you, thank you for being there through it all. I know you prayed for me, and I felt those prayers while I was going through my situation. You all helped me grow, and I appreciate you for being a part of my journey.

Last but definitely not least, Mom and Dad.

Dad, over the years we had some tough obstacles in front of us. Although through those challenges I learned the meaning of consequences.

You've always taught us to look at ourselves before placing blame on anyone else. I can hear your voice now, "Now Sade, you know that's not right." For that, I thank you. I realize that I will always be your baby girl. The one you got up early with to fix the famous "grits and eggs," the one who couldn't go to sleep without laying on your belly, the one who traveled everywhere you went because I wanted to be with my Dad. I love you so much.

Mom, my heart, the true definition of a friend. I love you to the ends. I know I was your last child and with me you woud've appreciated a manual. But, you never gave up on me. Thank You.

You taught us that even our struggle produces a future. You taught me how to be a mom, how to cook, how to clean, how to want more for my life. How to never let any man define who I am. You showed me what second chances look like. As much as I want to be the best mom, I know that your cape can never be cloned. I love you so much.

About the Author

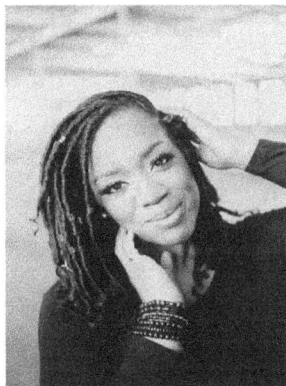

Fanchon Jackson was born in Spartanburg, South Carolina. She is a mother of four girls, one deceased (Grace Star).

Fanchon's desire to read and write started at a young age, as she was a part of several book clubs.

After her divorce, Fanchon became determined to heal mentally, physically, and spiritually, and her childhood passion of reading and writing became a place of healing.

This book entails a part of her story. It's a story of survival, endurance, and commitment, even in dark times.

Her ultimate goal is to help others see their self worth, knowing that they (YOU) matter in the end.

Motivated to live an "abundant life" (John 10:10), Fanchon, continues to keep God first, knowing everything else will follow.

www.ingramcontent.com/pod-product-compliance
Lightning Source LLC
Chambersburg PA
CBHW062119040426
42336CB00041B/2099